# Vitamins

Rhoda Nottridge

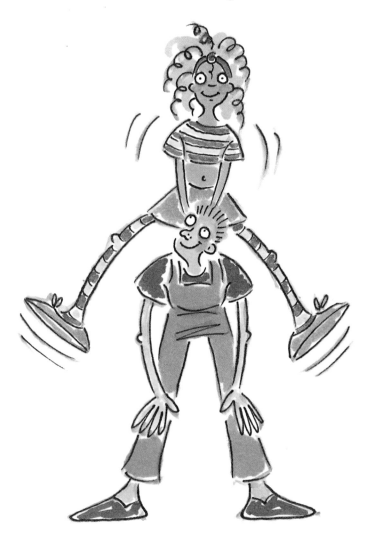

Wayland

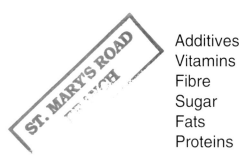

Additives
Vitamins
Fibre
Sugar
Fats
Proteins

Words printed in **bold** can be found in the glossary on page 30.

First published in 1992 by Wayland (Publishers) Ltd.
61 Western Road, Hove, East Sussex BN3 1JD

British Library Cataloguing in Publication Data

Nottridge, Rhoda
  Vitamins. – (Food Facts)
  I. Title II. Series
  612.399
  ISBN 0 7502 0359 5

© Copyright 1992 Wayland (Publishers) Ltd

*Series Editor:* Kathryn Smith
*Designer:* Helen White
*Artwork:* John Yates
*Cartoons:* Maureen Jackson

Typesetting by White Design
Printed and bound in Belgium by Casterman S.A.

# Contents

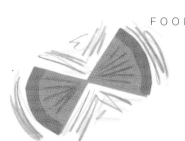

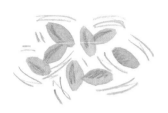

# What is a vitamin?

Imagine your body is like a machine. You need different fuels to keep the machine running smoothly. These important fuels include vitamins and minerals. We need them to help us stay healthy, grow and keep fit.

*OPPOSITE*
The shells, or husks, of brown rice are rich in vitamin B1

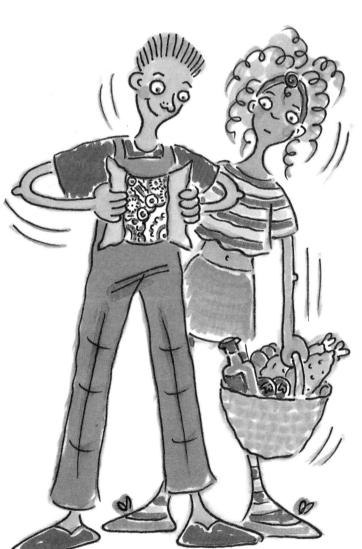

The first part of the word vitamin comes from the Latin language. In Latin, 'vita' means life. Vitamins are so called because it would be impossible to live without them.

**A great discovery**

Of course, vitamins have always been in food in very tiny amounts. But it was not until 1911 that a Polish scientist called Casimir Funk discovered the first vitamin.

When rice is polished (as a way of making it ready to eat) the outside shells are removed. Funk carried out experiments on some of these shells and discovered that there was something in them that could cure a very serious disease called beriberi. He realized that he had managed to **isolate** the first vitamin. This vitamin is now known as vitamin B1.

The discovery of other vitamins followed quickly. All around the world scientists began to find and name the different vitamins we know today, after the letters of the alphabet.

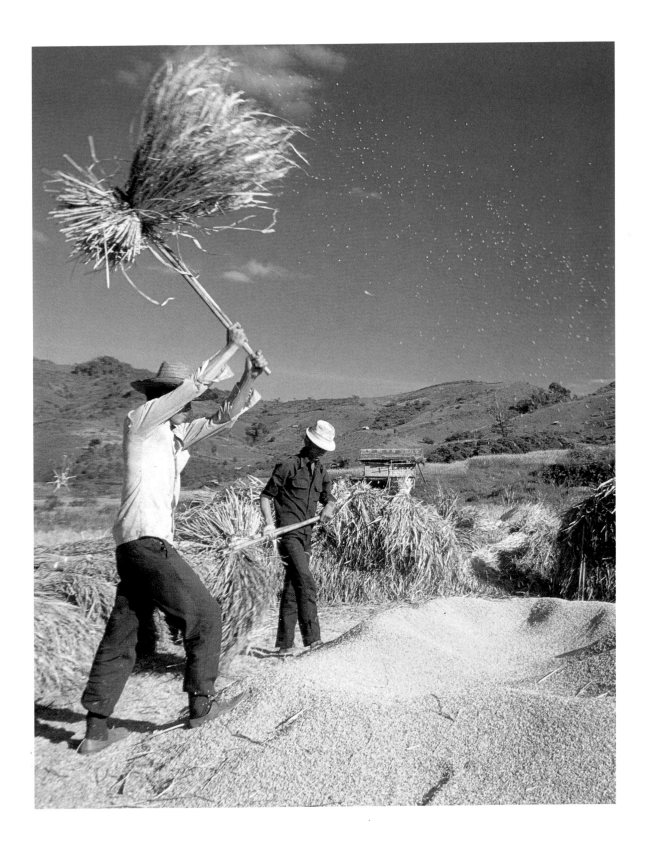

# Vitamins in the past

Vitamins are not all found in the same foods. For example, citrus fruits such as oranges, lemons and limes contain a lot of vitamin C, but no vitamin E.

### Vitamin c

As early as 1753 people knew that something in citrus fruit stopped sailors from getting a nasty disease called scurvy. During long sea voyages sailors often ate no fruit or vegetables, which contain important vitamins, for months. Doctors realized that there was something in citrus fruit which cured scurvy. However, in discovering this, some dreadful mistakes were made. Some doctors thought that it might be the **acidity** or sour taste in citrus fruit that stopped scurvy. They experimented by

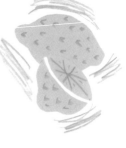

*BELOW* When they ripen these lemons will be an excellent source of vitamin C.

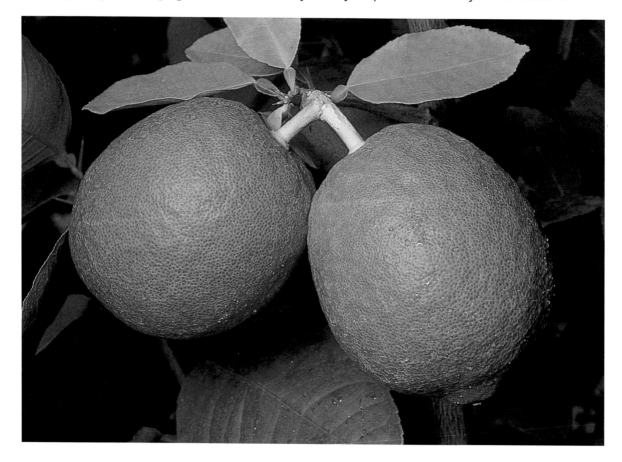

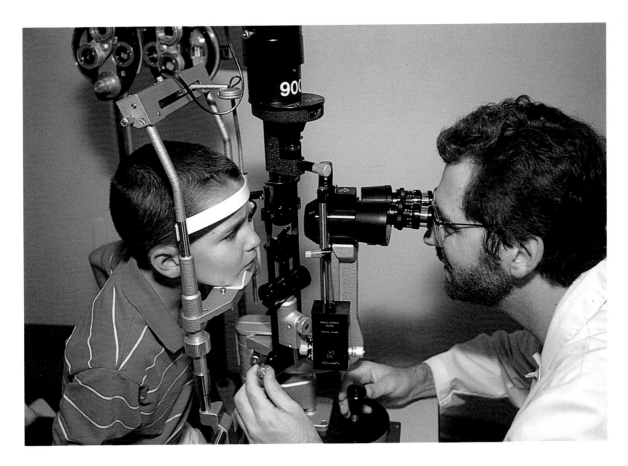

*ABOVE* Today, people with poor eyesight can have their eyes tested for glasses.

giving sailors large amounts of vinegar and other acidic things. This certainly did not cure the sailors' illness. Instead, it burned their stomachs!

When it was realized that citrus fruit cured scurvy, all ships in the British Navy were ordered to carry a supply of lemons and limes. The sailors ate some of the fruit every day to stop themselves from becoming ill with scurvy. Soon British sailors became known as 'limeys', after the limes.

## Vitamin A

In Greek and Roman times, people ate liver and cod liver oil to stop themselves from getting an illness called night blindness. The sufferer has poor eyesight and cannot see anything in the dark. But it was not until the late nineteenth century that doctors really began to investigate the relationship between food and eyesight.

In Brazil, in South America, people who were forced to work as slaves on **plantations** were found to have very bad eyesight. In 1883, a doctor realized this was because the slaves were never given any green vegetables to eat.

The vitamin that prevents poor eyesight is vitamin A. It was finally discovered by scientists in the USA, who found it in egg yolks and butter. By 1930 scientists had learned how to make it using chemicals.

## The B vitamins

In 1915 a disease called pellagra was so common on the slave plantations of the southern states of the USA, that doctors decided to investigate the mystery. Dr Joseph Goldberger was sent to a plantation to try and find out why so many of the slaves became ill with pellagra. He discovered that the slaves were only given corn bread, grain and fatty meat to eat. Because their **diets** were so bad, the slaves did not get any of the vitamin which would have stopped them from becoming ill. It was not until 1937 that the vitamin was named as vitamin B3.

There are several B vitamins, each one with a different number after it to

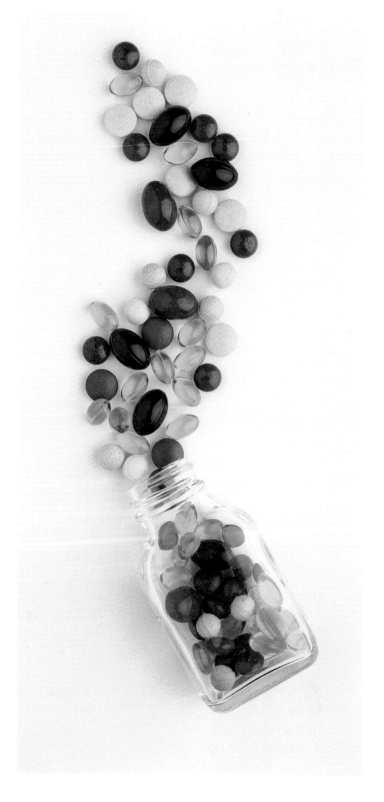

show which one it is. The name for all the B vitamins together is B complex.

### Vitamin D

Since the 1890s doctors thought that something in sunlight might stop people from getting a disease called rickets. This disease softens the bones so that sufferers have bow legs or knock-knees. The doctors knew that children who lived in countries with lots of sunshine did not get the disease.

It was also known that something in cod liver oil cured rickets in dogs. For a long time doctors were confused. Cod liver oil contained vitamin A. Yet other substances containing vitamin A did not cure rickets. Finally they realized that there was another vitamin in cod liver oil which was also found in sunlight. This vitamin cured rickets and was named vitamin D.

One by one, the vitamins we know today were discovered in different foods. Scientists then had to learn how to make these vitamins from chemicals, instead of taking them out of foods.

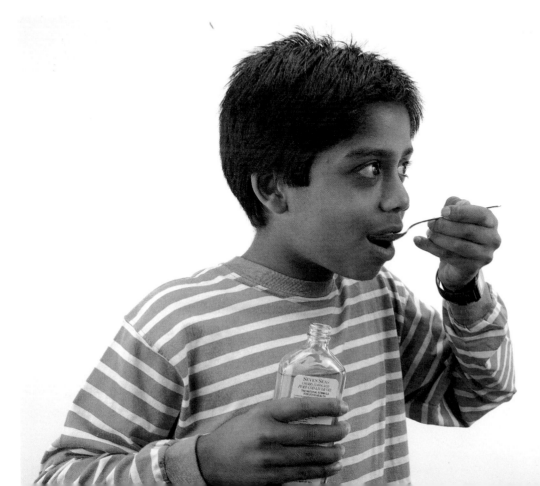

# Vitamin A : the sight vitamin

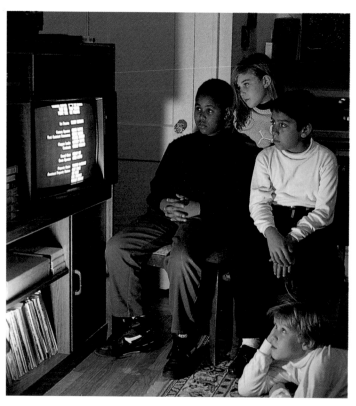

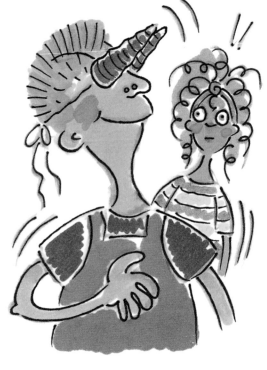

*ABOVE* Watching TV in a darkened room uses up a lot of vitamin A.

Vitamin A is often called the sight vitamin because it can help some people with sight problems. Those who have difficulty seeing in the dark or have problems seeing clearly when the light changes may need more vitamin A.

Itching eyes, styes and rough patches of skin can all suggest that more of this vitamin is needed. However, vitamin A does not only help our eyes. Together, vitamins A and E help to protect our bodies against air pollution. Like vitamin D, vitamin A is vital for the growth of bones and teeth. It also helps us recover from illnesses faster.

The idea that eating carrots helps us to see in the dark is actually true. Carrots contain something called carotene, which is a yellowish colouring, rich in vitamin A. It is also

**Science Corner**

Some vitamins are known by a full name rather than a letter or number. We need to be able to recognize these names in order to know exactly what the food we eat contains.

To help you learn to recognize them, look on the outside of food packets. There are often tables showing **nutritional information.** Cereal boxes are a good place to start looking.

Copy the chart below and fill it in, writing down where you found each of the vitamins.

| | Ascorbic acid | Folic acid | Niacin | Riboflavin | Thiamin |
|---|---|---|---|---|---|
| | ( Vit C) | (B Group) | (B Group) | (B Group) | (B Group) |
| Where it is found | lemon barley water | | Cornflakes | Cornflakes | Cornflakes |
| '' | | | | | |
| '' | | | | | |
| '' | | | | | |
| '' | | | | | |

found in most dark green or yellow vegetables and fruit, such as parsley, marrows, apricots, oranges, peaches and melons. Fish liver oils, milk and butter are also good sources of vitamin A.

Some vitamins such as vitamin A stay in the body for a long time. We need to eat food containing others all the time, because the body does not store them up for use when it needs them.

# The B vitamins

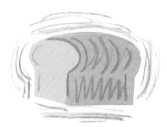

There are thirteen different types of vitamins in the B group. Together they are known as B complex. There are three main ones: vitamins B1, B2 and B3. They work together to look after the health of our **nervous system**, skin and **digestion**.

The B vitamins can be very easily damaged. Up to half of the B vitamins in food are destroyed by heat during cooking. However, it is not only strong heat which can destroy them. Milk which has been left in the sun loses as much as three-quarters of its vitamin B2 in three hours.

Brewer's yeast, wheatgerm and cereals which have not been **processed** contain more vitamin B1 than any other substance.

Milk and liver are the only foods which contain a large amount of vitamin B2.

Vitamin B3 is found in liver, meat with little fat on it, fish, brewer's yeast and wheat-germ. This is an important vitamin because it helps the brain work properly.

One of the most recently-discovered vitamins is B12.

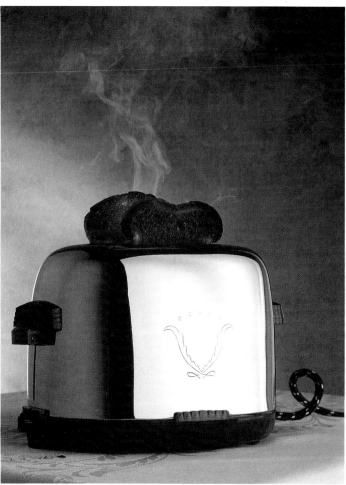

*ABOVE* A piece of bread loses one-third of its vitamin B1 when it is toasted.

It was not found until 1948. It is vital for keeping our blood and nerves healthy. **Vegetarians** need to take extra care that they get enough of it. This is because although B12 is found in meat, especially liver and kidneys, very few plants contain any of it.

However, there are two Japanese seaweeds which contain a lot of vitamin B12. They are called wakame and kombu. These can be bought from health food shops and can be used in many delicious recipes. The body stores this vitamin for as long as three years, so we do not need to eat it everyday.

Eating green leafy vegetables gives us another important B vitamin which is called folic acid. It is also found in liver, kidney and brewer's yeast. Folic acid is needed to make our blood and to keep the brain healthy. It is very important that pregnant women and young children get enough of this vitamin.

## Science Corner

Bean shoots are an excellent source of vitamins. They contain not only vitamin C, but many of the other important vitamins too.

   Why not add bean shoots to your diet by growing them from beans? You can eat the shoots when they are just a few centimetres long.
1. You will need half a cupful of green mung beans (you can buy these from a health food shop) and a jam jar. Soak the beans overnight in water.  2. Then drain off the water and place the beans in a covered jam jar in a warm, dark place.  3. Rinse and drain the beans twice a day with warm water.  4. In just a few days time the shoots will be about 5 cm long and ready to eat.

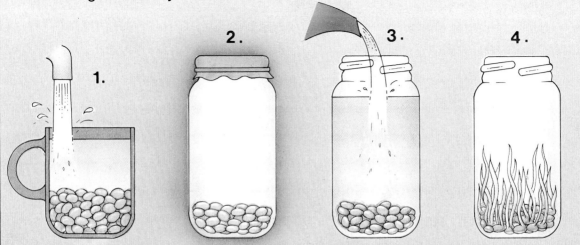

# Vitamin C: the cold cure ?

Most animals make vitamin c in their bodies. Apes, guinea pigs and humans are different. They have to get vitamin c from the food they eat.

Vitamin c is very useful. It helps to heal cuts, bruises and burns. It is important for the growth and health of our teeth, gums, blood and bones. One of its most important functions is to help the body fight against illnesses.

*BELOW* Eating an orange is a quick and easy way of getting vitamin c.

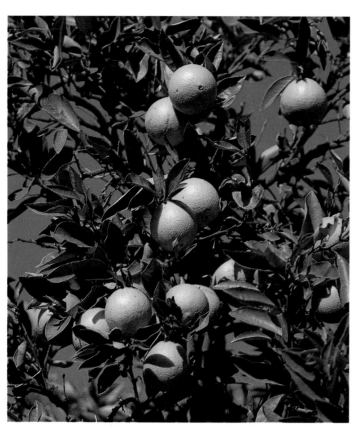

Citrus fruit, berries, green peppers and tomatoes contain a large amount of vitamin c. Fresh bean sprouts are especially rich in vitamin c. Half a cupful contains the same amount as six glasses of orange juice. The older food becomes, the less vitamin c it contains. This is because vitamin c disappears over time. A newly-dug potato will contain three times as much vitamin c as a potato that has been stored for the winter.

Vitamin c dissolves in water, so that most of the vitamin c in fruit and vegetables is lost when they are cooked.

Some scientists believe that we can stop ourselves from getting colds and cure them by taking large doses of vitamin c.

We cannot be sure if this is true, but our bodies do need more vitamin c when we are ill. This is because the body uses up vitamin c fighting illnesses.

We do not really know how much vitamin c our bodies need. However, we do know that the body does not store it, so we need to make sure that we get some every day.

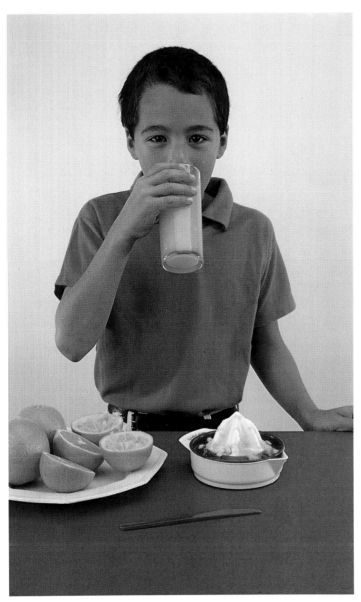

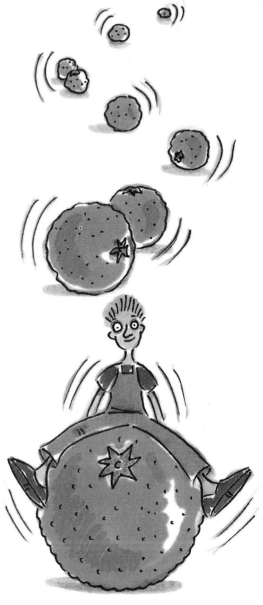

ABOVE Freshly squeezed orange juice is a healthy and delicious alternative to processed soft drinks.

In most countries a government health department tells us how much of each vitamin it thinks we need each day. The amount of vitamin C that is suggested differs in many countries. In Britain a dose of 30 mg for an adult and 20 mg for a child is suggested. Other countries such as the USA and the USSR suggest much higher doses. Although large amounts of vitamin C are not dangerous, experiments show that our bodies do not like to be overloaded with it.

## Vitamin c Drink

Many fruit drinks you can buy at the shops have been processed. This means that many of the vitamins the fruit contains have been destroyed. Why not make your own delicious lemon drink which is full of vitamin c?

### You will need
4 fresh lemons
3/4 litre of cold water
Sugar (to taste)

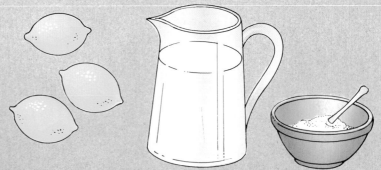

1. Cut the lemons in half and squeeze them over a jug until all the juice is squeezed out. 2. Take care to remove all the pips! 3. Dissolve a little sugar in a small amount of hot water and add to the lemon juice. 4. Add the cold water and stir, to mix the ingredients. 5. Chill the drink in the fridge for at least one hour. It is now ready to drink.

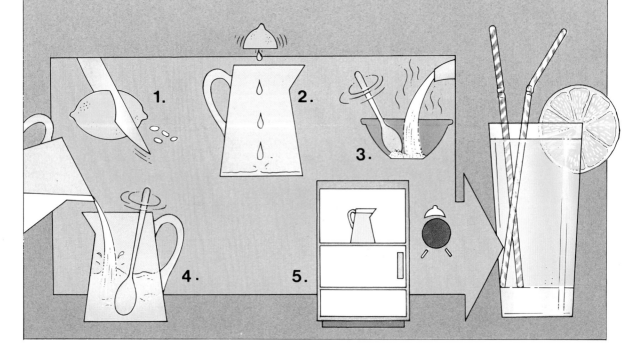

# Vitamin D: the sunshine vitamin

Vitamin D is only found in small amounts in a few foods such as eggs, butter and oily fish. Cod liver oil, which also contains vitamin A, is the best source.

Vitamin D is often called the sunshine vitamin, because we can get it from sunlight. When the sun shines on the oils found on our bare skin, vitamin D is made. If we swim or have a bath before going out in the sun, less or no vitamin D is made. This is because many of the oils on our skin are washed off by water.

People who live in countries where there is not much sunlight, such as Britain, may not get enough vitamin D. The elderly, disabled or sick (who may be indoors a lot) often do not get enough of the sunshine vitamin. People who live in countries where there is a lot of sunshine rarely have this problem.

Without vitamin D children can get diseases of the bones such as rickets. This painful illness causes deformed bones. In the 1900s rickets was common in Europe. But since the discovery of vitamin D few people have rickets. A good supply of vitamin D will also help to keep our teeth strong and healthy.

People with darker skins have more protection against the sun's rays, but absorb less sunlight. So people with dark skin living in countries which get little sunshine, need to take special care that they get enough vitamin D.

*BELOW* Although sunshine helps us make vitamin D, we need to protect our skin from the sun's strong rays by wearing suntan lotion.

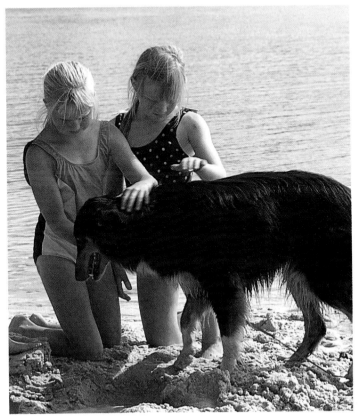

# Vitamin E: the miracle vitamin?

Vitamin E was first found in wheatgerm oil in 1936. It has become famous as a 'miracle' cure for all sorts of things, although no one really knows what it does.

People in the USA discovered that if they put vitamin E on scars and wrinkles they seemed to fade away a little. Some people thought that if they used enough vitamin E on their skin, they would look young forever! Although creams containing vitamin E cannot make skin young again, it does help to heal burns and scars if it is used immediately.

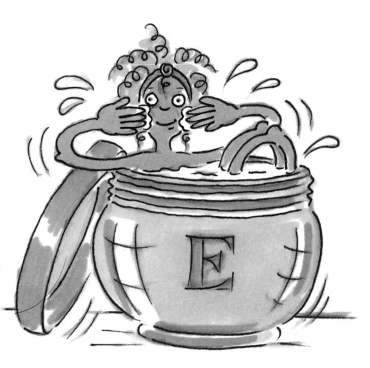

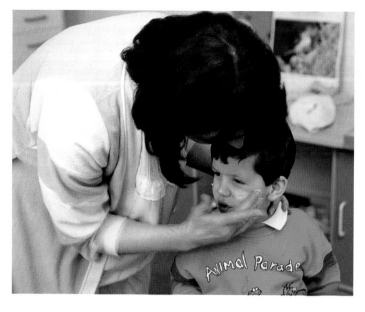

*LEFT* This little boy uses vitamin E cream to help cure his eczema.

People who have heart diseases and problems with circulation can also be helped by taking large doses of vitamin E.

In addition, vitamin E protects our lungs from air pollution. It also protects the vitamin A in our bodies and helps to store it longer.

## Looking Good with Vitamins

Vitamins are as important to helping us look good as they are to our health.

Look carefully at this chart. Now think about your own body. Do you have strong nails? Are your teeth healthy? Is your hair shining? Do you think you are getting enough of these five vitamins to keep healthy and look good?

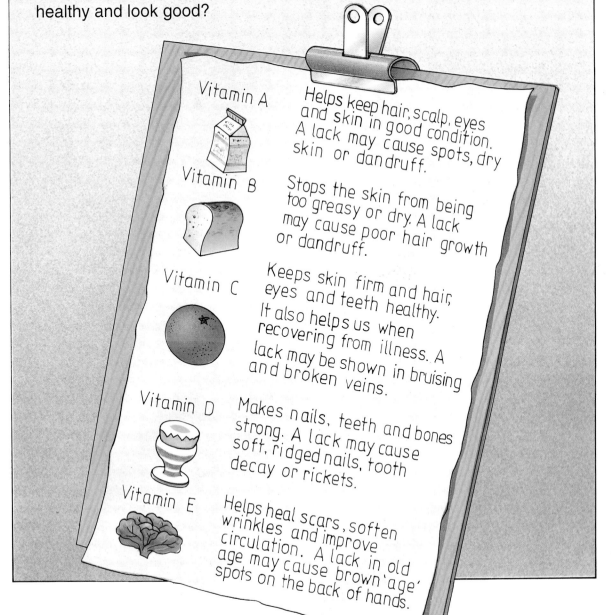

Vitamin A — Helps keep hair, scalp, eyes and skin in good condition. A lack may cause spots, dry skin or dandruff.

Vitamin B — Stops the skin from being too greasy or dry. A lack may cause poor hair growth or dandruff.

Vitamin C — Keeps skin firm and hair, eyes and teeth healthy. It also helps us when recovering from illness. A lack may be shown in bruising and broken veins.

Vitamin D — Makes nails, teeth and bones strong. A lack may cause soft, ridged nails, tooth decay or rickets.

Vitamin E — Helps heal scars, soften wrinkles and improve circulation. A lack in old age may cause brown 'age' spots on the back of hands.

# How many more vitamins ?

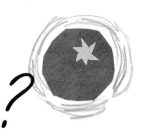

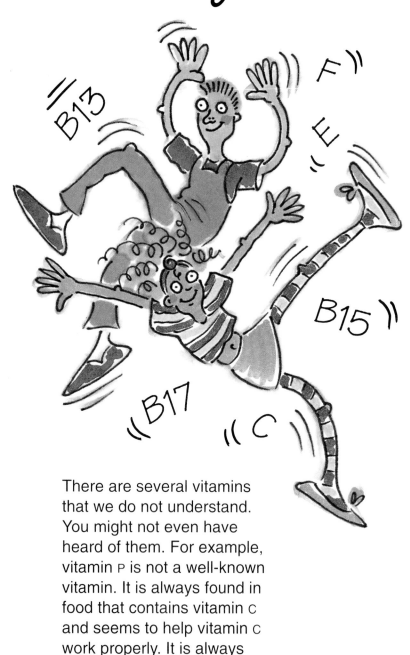

Vitamin F is always found alongside vitamin E and is needed, among other things, to keep skin healthy. It is found in vegetable oils and cereals, but is easily destroyed when food is processed.

When we cut ourselves, our blood forms a scab to stop us from bleeding. Vitamin K helps blood to make scabs. It is quite easy to get enough vitamin K, as it is found in many foods. These include greens, tomatoes, honey, egg yolk, bran, some cereals and wheatgerm.

Many people know very little about some B vitamins, such as B13, B15 and B17. Although you may not have heard of it, B15 is used a lot in the USSR. People believe it can help with skin and heart problems. However, **artificially**-made vitamin B15 might not be safe for use. More tests need to be done in order to find out what it really does. Scientists also need to do more tests on vitamin B17, which is found in the seeds of most fruits, as no one really knows much about it.

There are several vitamins that we do not understand. You might not even have heard of them. For example, vitamin P is not a well-known vitamin. It is always found in food that contains vitamin C and seems to help vitamin C work properly. It is always found in the **pulp** and **pith** of fruit.

Another vitamin has been found in raw cabbage, but scientists have not yet discovered how to make it using chemicals. This vitamin, named vitamin U, is thought to be able to help people who have ulcers.

*BELOW* Calcium helps to make our teeth strong but we need to clean them regularly to keep them healthy.

## Minerals

There are fifteen minerals needed by our bodies for healthy growth, repair and general well-being. We need minerals as well as vitamins because without them, our bodies cannot use vitamins.

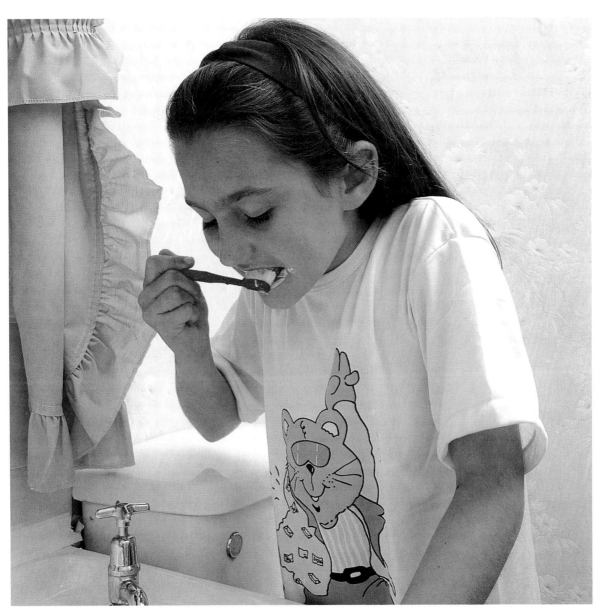

## Mineral Needs

Write down what you have eaten so far today. How many of these five minerals did your meals contain?

Can you think of other foods you could have eaten instead to make sure you had enough of all five minerals?

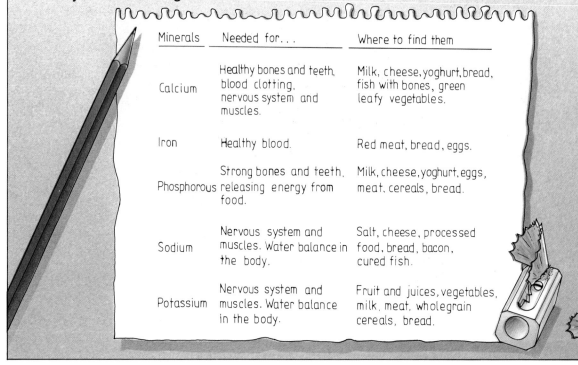

| Minerals | Needed for... | Where to find them |
|---|---|---|
| Calcium | Healthy bones and teeth, blood clotting, nervous system and muscles. | Milk, cheese, yoghurt, bread, fish with bones, green leafy vegetables. |
| Iron | Healthy blood. | Red meat, bread, eggs. |
| Phosphorous | Strong bones and teeth. releasing energy from food. | Milk, cheese, yoghurt, eggs, meat. cereals, bread. |
| Sodium | Nervous system and muscles. Water balance in the body. | Salt, cheese, processed food, bread, bacon, cured fish. |
| Potassium | Nervous system and muscles. Water balance in the body. | Fruit and juices, vegetables, milk, meat, wholegrain cereals, bread. |

Unfortunately our bodies cannot make minerals. So we must get a good supply from our food. The most important are calcium, phosphorus and magnesium, which help our bones and teeth grow and stay healthy. Iron, sodium and potassium are all needed for our blood. Our bodies contain enough iron to make a 5 cm nail!

Some minerals are only needed in very tiny amounts but are still very important. They are called trace elements and include copper, zinc, magnesium and fluorine.

# Vitamin supplements

There are two ways in which we can make sure that we get enough vitamins.

One is to make sure that we include all the foods that contain different vitamins in our diets. If this is not possible, the alternative is to take vitamin supplements.

*BELOW* Vitamin supplements can come in many different forms; drinks, pills, powders and liquids.

Since scientists discovered vitamins, they have found ways of making them artificially using chemicals or by **extracting** them from plants and animals. These vitamins are then put into pills, powders or liquids called supplements.

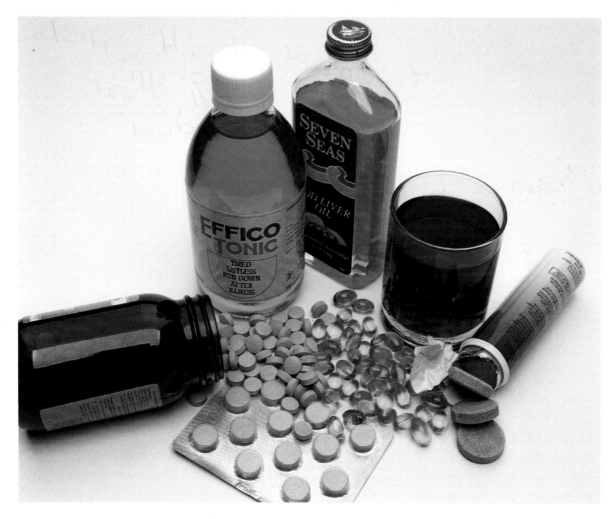

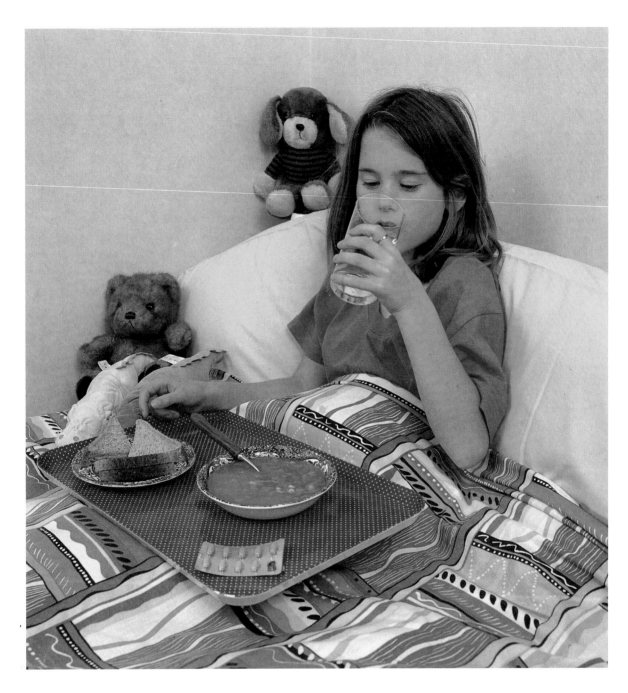

Vitamin and mineral supplements should not be taken instead of food. The body would not be able to use them without food as well.

*ABOVE* When ill, vitamin pills are a good way of making sure you get enough vitamins.

There may be certain times in our lives when vitamin supplements may be useful, such as when we are ill, or recovering from an illness.

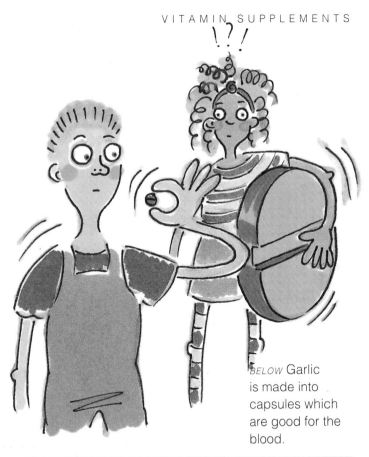

Some scientists and doctors have different ideas as to whether it is a good idea to take vitamin supplements. Some even feel that overloading our bodies with vitamins can be harmful. There are certainly some vitamins which we should not take in large **doses**, such as vitamins A and D.

The second problem with vitamins and minerals is how big a dose we should take. Most countries recommend a daily amount of the most important vitamins but these amounts vary in different countries.

Many supplements are sold which are made from foods which contain a lot of a particular vitamin or mineral. Some supplements contain many vitamins or minerals. For example, spirulina was first used by the ancient people the Aztecs of Mexico and can now be bought as pills or powder. It contains many vitamins and minerals.

Brewer's yeast was originally a yeast that came from beer-making. Today it can be bought as a powder and added to soups, stews or cereals. It is an excellent source of all the B vitamins.

*BELOW* Garlic is made into capsules which are good for the blood.

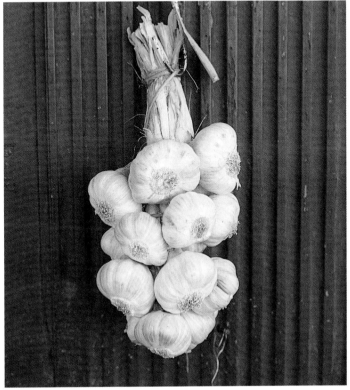

25

# What vitamins do you need?

Children and young people need to make sure that they get enough vitamins and minerals while they are growing. This will help to make sure that they grow strong and healthy.

Some groups of people need to take particular care. For example, teenage girls often do not get enough vitamins and minerals. They need to take special care that they get plenty of iron, vitamin A and vitamin B2. Calcium and vitamin D are also very important for all growing young people, as they are needed for the growth of strong bones.

People who enjoy doing a lot of sport also need to make sure they get enough vitamins to keep their strength up. The B vitamins may be particularly useful, because B1 is lost through sweating. Hard exercise also makes our bodies lose vitamin B2.

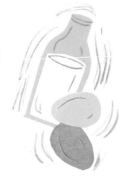

*BELOW* A healthy diet containing all the important vitamins will help you keep your body fit.

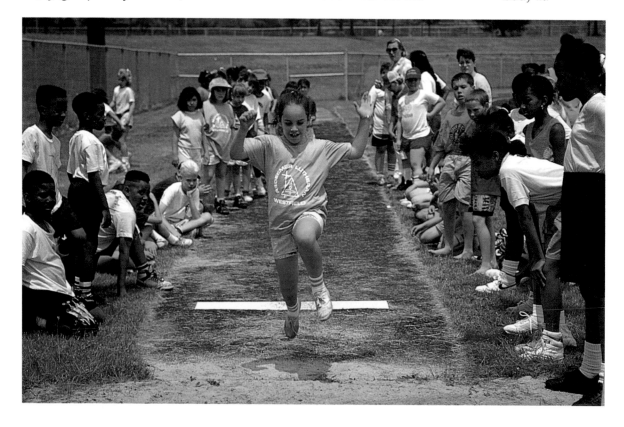

## Where to find Vitamins

This chart shows the best sources of the most important vitamins.
   Keep a record for a week of what you ate for breakfast, lunch and dinner. Use this chart to see how healthy your diet is. How many foods containing vitamin A did you eat? How many foods containing vitamin B1 did you eat?...and so on.

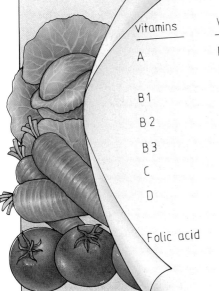

| Vitamins | Where to find them |
|---|---|
| A | Liver, kidney, oily fish, egg yolk, cabbage, margarine, butter, whole milk. |
| B1 | Bread, cereals, vegetables, milk, meat. |
| B2 | Milk, cheese, eggs, meat, green leafy vegetables. |
| B3 | Meat, fish, cheese, milk, bread. |
| C | Fruit, fresh and frozen vegetables. |
| D | Oily fish, eggs, margarine, wholemeal bread, nuts, green leafy vegetables. |
| Folic acid | Liver, kidney, green leafy vegetables, wholemeal bread, oranges and bananas. |

These vitamins cannot make us better sportspeople, but we will feel tired if we do not get enough of them. Getting enough vitamins makes our bodies work at their best.
   Elderly people may need extra vitamins because their bodies are slower at taking the vitamins out of food and because they eat less.
   Slimmers need to take care that they are getting plenty of vitamins. Eating less food means that you need to watch what you eat very carefully, in order to make sure you are not cutting out important vitamins.
   Cigarette smokers destroy the very vitamins in their bodies that are so important to their health. Just one cigarette destroys the amount of vitamin C that you need for one day.

# Getting vitamins from our food

If we eat a balanced diet we can make sure that we get all the vitamins we need from our food. However, much of the food we eat today is processed. When food is processed it often loses many of its vitamins and minerals. Frozen food keeps more of its vitamins than tinned or dried foods.

Vitamins can be destroyed in a number of ways. Light destroys vitamins A, B and C and air affects vitamins A and C. For this reason it is best to only prepare food when we are ready to cook and eat it. If food must be prepared early, the vitamin C in salads and fruit can be kept by sprinkling a little lemon juice on the food.

When we soak or cook fruit and vegetables in water a lot of the vitamins that food contain are lost. This is because some vitamins, such as B and C, dissolve in the water. It is better to **steam** fruit and vegetables than to cook them in water. We should also try to cook food for a shorter amount of time so that less goodness is lost.

*BELOW* Meals at fast food restaurants often contain highly processed foods.

Peeling fruit and vegetables also takes away vitamins as they are often found just below the skin. A potato loses around one-third of its vitamin C when it is peeled. However, fruit and vegetables must be washed well before we eat them if they are not peeled.

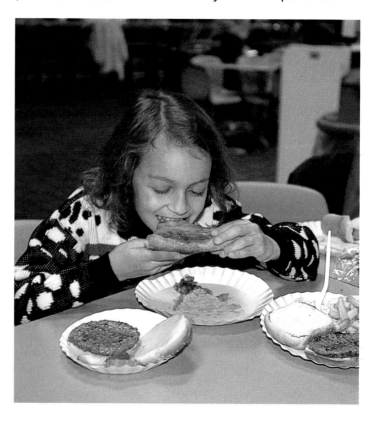

The main way in which we can help our bodies to stay fit and healthy is to eat a good variety of different fresh foods.

## Meal Planning

It is easy to read through a list of foods containing all the important vitamins. It is much harder to make sure the food you eat contains them all!

 With a friend, plan a menu for either breakfast, lunch or dinner. Try to make sure that the meal contains as many of the vitamins and minerals necessary for good health as possible. Use the tables on pages 22 and 27 to help you.

 The menu below suggests what a healthy lunch might look like.

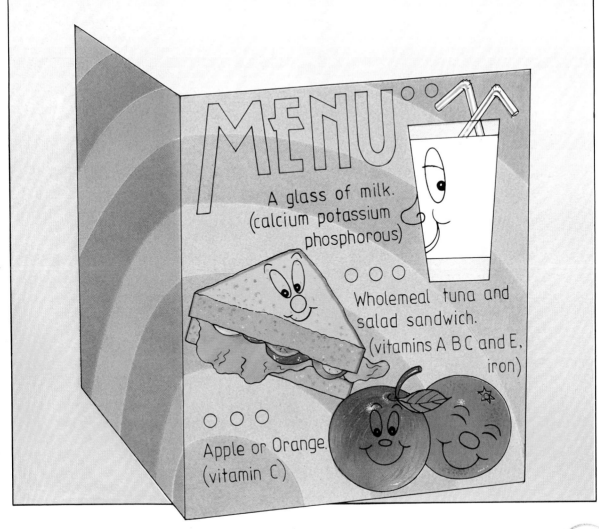

MENU

A glass of milk.
(calcium potassium phosphorous)

Wholemeal tuna and salad sandwich.
(vitamins A B C and E, iron)

Apple or Orange.
(vitamin C)

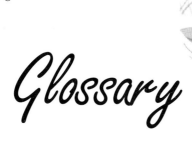

# Glossary

**Acidity**  How acid or sour something is. Vinegar has a sharp, sour taste because it is acidic.

**Artificially**  When something does not occur naturally, but is made by people.

**Diet**  Our diet is made up of all the things we eat.

**Digestion**  When the body changes the food we eat into its many different parts. These many parts may include vitamins and minerals.

**Doses**  Certain amounts of something, taken at regular times of the day. Medicine is taken in doses.

**Extracting**  Removing or separating something from the things it is joined to.

**Isolate**  To find something on its own.

**Nervous system**  The part of the body which is made up of all our nerves.

**Nutritional Information**  Information on a food packet about what vitamins, minerals and other nutrients the food contains.

**Pith**  The soft white lining inside fruit such as oranges.

**Plantations**  Large farms where the land has been cleared to grow one type of crop only.

**Processed**  When food has been changed by adding new things and taking others away.

**Pulp**  The fleshy, soft part of a fruit or plant. The pulp of an apple is the  part you eat.

**Steam**  Cooking vegetables in a container above boiling water, so that the vegetables cook by steam rather than being in the water.

**Vegetarians**  People who eat no meat from animals.

# Books to read

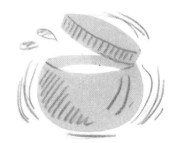

*Diet* by Brian Ward (Franklin Watts, 1991)

*Food Fun Book* by Rosemary Stanton (Hamlyn, 1988)

*Healthy Eating* by Wayne Jackman (Wayland, 1990)

*Thinking about Food* by Ralph Whitlock (Lutterworth, 1980)

**For teachers**

*The Vitamin Fact Finder* by Carol Hunter (Thorsons, 1987)

*The Vitamin Bible* by Earl Mindell (Arlington Books, 1982)

**Picture Acknowledgements**
Bruce Coleman 6; Chapel Studio *Cover*, 8, 9, 23, 24; Eye Ubiquitous 21;
J. Greenberg 10, 26, 28; Tony Stone 5, 12, 14, 25; Zefa 7.

# Index

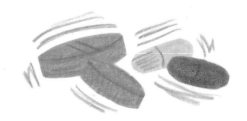